THE ART OF COACHING

Dan John

ISBN: 978-1-963675-15-3 (paperback)

Published by OS Press

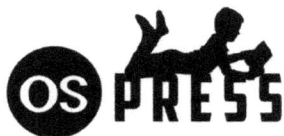

Table of Contents

Dedication

I grew a bit emotional when I reread the story of my dad spending hours with me out on the field at South City High. It struck me that he never had the chance to read my books and articles on athletics — books I know he would have loved.

Now, as I approach an age older than he ever lived to see, I find myself thinking often of Dylan Thomas:

And you, my father, there on the sad height,
Curse, bless, me now with your fierce tears, I pray.
Do not go gentle into that good night.
Rage, rage against the dying of the light.

To Albert Lewis John. For you, Dad.

And… to the friends we lost on that terrible August day.

Introduction

During the pandemic lockdown—one of the strangest and hardest stretches of my life—I organized a series of free online lectures through danjohnuniversity.com. With the help of Brian Gwaltney, we posted hours of workshops on a wide range of topics, from fat loss to the philosophy of coaching.

It was a simple idea: give people something to think about (and maybe laugh about) while the world seemed to be going sideways.

Afterward, people kept asking—through emails, workshops, and in person—if I'd ever write out these talks in a way that captured all the little details that inevitably get lost in a one-hour presentation.

The truth is, *The Art of Coaching* started long before all that. It began as a three-day, in-person workshop… back when people still traveled, booked hotels, and sat shoulder to shoulder listening to some guy with a marker and a whiteboard. I wanted to publish this material for those who couldn't attend.

Then, of course, the workshops ended—another casualty of the epidemic. Most of my clients and readers, understandably, weren't asking for lectures on assessment models. They needed practical workouts they could do with minimal equipment and limited time. So, I put together resources like the Armor Building Formula and Easy Strength for Fat Loss to help keep people moving (and sane).

Still, *The Art of Coaching* never left my mind. It's the framework I use not just for training athletes, but also for teaching, parenting, and steering through life's inevitable messes. It's about saying "both/and" instead of getting stuck in "either/or." It's about keeping the client—or the athlete, student, or anyone you're trying to help—moving toward a clear goal, while constantly adjusting for life's surprises.

I've been coaching since 1979. In that time, I've learned that success isn't about perfect plans. It's about having a compass you can trust and the willingness to keep checking it, no matter how many times the winds change.

So that's what this book is: part philosophy, part toolbox, part honest stories from someone who's tried nearly everything—sometimes twice, just to make sure it was a bad idea. My hope is that it helps you, whether you're a coach, teacher, parent, or simply someone trying to move from one place to another.

Chapter One

Coaching: The BIG Picture

Like many coaches I know, I'm not a big fan of watching sports *as a fan*. Now, don't get me wrong—I *love* sports. But as the old saying goes (often attributed to Albert Einstein and maybe a dozen others), *"I love humanity—it's people I can't stand."* That's kind of how I feel about fans.

Whether I'm in stadium seats, a bar, or someone's living room, there's always that person nearby—the one who finds fatal flaws in every play, every call, every coaching decision. It's exhausting.

Years ago, I developed a straightforward approach to explaining the levels of coaching. It's a lot like being funny.

Level One: Telling a Joke

This is the "chicken-crossing-the-road" tier. A setup, a punchline, a few chuckles, and everyone goes back to what they were doing.

Level Two: Stand-Up Set

Now you're talking. I once took a four-day stand-up comedy workshop that ended with five minutes on stage in front of a very drunk crowd. It was tough. Now imagine tacking on 55 more minutes and trying to *stay funny*. It's hard work. That's coaching at a deeper level—holding attention, reading the room, adjusting on the fly.

Level Three: The Entertainer

Think Gene Kelly. Or for modern audiences, Hugh Jackman or Hannah Waddingham. These are people who can make you laugh, sing their heart out, charm you on a talk show, and then deliver a monologue that leaves you breathless.

Steve Martin can go from riffing with Martin Short to ripping on a banjo with his band.

That's master-level work.

The typical fan? They're Level One—if we're being generous. They parrot what the talking heads said on the pregame show and question the toughness of an athlete limping off the field.

My goal is to help you pull back the curtain—to think, act, and grow like a coach.

Let me say this (again, if you've ever heard me speak):

The word **"coach"** originally referred to a four-wheeled carriage that took someone from **here** to **there**. That's our job—to move people forward.

And most of the time, coaching is simply ensuring people stay *in* the vehicle.

Don't let them leap off to chase every shiny object that zips by the window.

Honestly, coaching often feels like that message you hear at amusement parks:

"Please keep your hands, arms, feet, and legs inside the ride at all times."

Let's start from here. Let's see where we can go.

I often tell attendees at my workshops that one of the best starting points for coaches isn't a training manual or a biomechanics textbook—it's the book *"Think Like a Freak"* by Steven Levitt and Stephen Dubner (yes, the *Freakonomics* guys).

It's technically a book about economics, but it's *really* about better thinking. It offers tools that every coach should carry, including these two game-changers:

1. "Knowing What to Measure Simplifies Life."

As a throws coach, if the discus goes farther, I'm *right*.
As a strength coach, if the bar gets heavier, I'm *right*.
As a fat loss coach, if the waistline drops, I'm *right*.

If you manage a sales team and one person outsells everyone else combined, I don't need a think tank to tell me—they're *right*.

Clarity comes from choosing the right metrics.

2. "Don't Fear the Obvious."

Want to get stronger?

Lift weights.

I've been saying that since 1965, and people still lean in, waiting for "the real secret."

Here it is—the greatest secret I've learned in over five decades:

There are no secrets.

Tired? Sleep.

Thirsty? Drink water.

Weak? Lift weights.

Don't overcomplicate what doesn't need to be complicated.

Steno and Tensive Symbols and The Art of Communicating (in Coaching)

There's a story about Gary Player, the great golfer, which may or may not be true. Honestly, I don't care, but I was able to ask him about it in the Delta Sky Club in Atlanta (it's "true enough," he said, holding his chicken noodle soup).

After a particularly rough round, a fan shouted, **"I'd trade my best day for your worst day!"**

According to the story, Player—who is not exactly an imposing figure—walked over and snapped:

"No, you wouldn't. You wouldn't get up before sunrise to practice putting, then hit drives until your hands bleed and your skin peels from sunburn. You just want a good game. You don't want to earn one."

It took me a while to truly appreciate that sentiment.

In Track and Field or American Football, people generally understand that no one rolls out of bed and pole vaults 19 feet or plays linebacker in the Super Bowl. You don't snatch 300 pounds or clean 400 pounds without years—if not decades—of effort.

However, in the world of strength and conditioning, especially within the fitness industry, everyone wants shortcuts. We used to joke about "weekend wonders"—people who attend a two-day cert and emerge as experts in kettlebells, Olympic lifting, gymnastics, nutrition, and programming.

Why waste years when you can "learn it all" in a weekend?

Especially within the fitness industry, everyone wants shortcuts.

Today, we can string together a few scientific-sounding words and build a cult-like following. Sometimes I look at this industry and fall to my knees, praying people can see through the nonsense. But it's tough. We all fall into a trap, and the best way I can explain it is to borrow from Shakespeare: words, words, words.

Whenever you teach something new, you run into two major barriers. Every word, every symbol, every concept carries baggage. Ludwig Wittgenstein clarified this long ago, but in fitness and performance, we deal with it daily.

There are two types of symbols: **steno** and **tensive**.

- **Steno symbols** have one clear meaning. (To remember: spell it backward—"ONEts.")
- **Tensive symbols** depend on context.

A **desk** is a steno symbol. No one says, "She's so *desk*." It just means desk.

"Bad," however, is a tensive symbol:

"That was a bad movie."
"That movie was *bad*!"

Is it good or bad? It depends on the tone and context. "Dog" is another:

"Watch out for him—he's a dog."
"We worked like dogs."
"I'm dog tired."

Once, my vet said she couldn't clip my dog's nails because he was "crocodiling." I still don't know how my house pet turned into an ancient reptile, but I understood the point.

For most fat loss clients, **"diet"** and **"exercise"** are steno symbols:

- **Diet** = starvation, rabbit food, suffering, self-loathing.
- **Exercise** = sweat, pain, vomit, and more suffering.

So if I say,

"Let's learn to shop smarter, cook nutritious meals, and treat food as fuel...",

they hear:
"Rabbit food. Starvation. Sadness."

If I say,

"We're going to teach you to move better so you feel, look, and live better...",

they hear:
"Sweat. Pain. Vomit."

The media reinforces this. Ads promise to shred, melt, or punish fat. Diets claim to detox or purge you into shape. TV shows and magazines peddle unrealistic timelines and masochistic methods. So "diet" and "training" become fixed symbols of misery.

To counter this, we must first help clients realize they're operating under **unexamined steno symbols.** We then offer an alternative: a sensible approach to nutrition and movement. It takes time. It takes trust.

I know this because I lived it.

My career in the discus helped me become a better strength coach. But for years, I had my own steno symbol:

Coaching, training, and success = Nose to the grindstone until it rubs off.

And I was wrong.

What actually works? **Quality practice. Over years.**

If you asked me for the "secret"—the fitness version of "buy low, sell high"—I'd whisper:

Be outstanding in your field.

And yes, I mean literally:

You're going to spend a lot of time *out standing in a field.*

One of my favorite memories is of my father, Big Al John—all 112 pounds of him—standing at the 180-foot mark, waiting to stop and return my discus throws. They'd hit the ground and skid out to 200 or 220 feet. He'd flip one up with his foot and throw it back... maybe 20 feet.

Then he'd jog after it in his tie and slacks and toss it another 20 feet.

At the time, I'd get frustrated. If I'd just run out there, I could have cut down on the dozens of "Big Al throws." But today, I'd trade almost anything for one more minute, one more throw, one more walk across that field with my dad. I only recently appreciated the biggest insight: I got better because my dad was "out standing" out there with me!

Lesson #1 of performance in any domain: You must be out there.

You can't rush it. You can't fake it. You've got to put in the time, energy, and patience.

If you want to make 10,000 throws a year, you've got to live "out there."

These days, I see fitness influencers brag about their "15 months of coaching experience," and I think… wow. The level of hubris. My first article wasn't published until after I underwent multiple surgeries, spent thousands of hours under the bar, and had enough time coaching to fill a dozen résumés.

When I meet the best in the field, I'm always struck by how much they've tested, discarded, refined, and relearned.

It takes time.

Chapter Two

The Art of Coaching

Coaching is both a science and an art. I think of it like being a chef: you have a recipe, but you still need to work with what you have on hand. The ingredients change depending on where you are, who you're coaching, and what's available. You adapt, adjust, and—sometimes—improvise.

There's nothing wrong with following a proven program. But you'll rarely find that what worked in one environment transfers perfectly to another. Good coaching is more than instruction—it's *translation*. It's the dance between a client's goals and their current reality, assessed continuously and compassionately.

Coaching is most effective when it is done by understanding the goal and assessing continuously.

Percy Cerutty once said:

"The teachings of the coach must always be suspect when he attempts to develop techniques based upon theories worked out intellectually. Unless he gets the idea from personal experience and feelings first, he is most likely to be wrong in principle."

Coaching starts in the trenches. Theory matters, but it must be tested against reality. That's why my view is simple:

Coaching is most effective when it is done by understanding the goal and assessing continuously. That's the art.

Defining the Art of Coaching

Throughout my careers as a teacher, administrator, coach, professor, and parent, I've realized something: the idea of "either/or" might work well for ultimatums, but it's a poor lens for working with actual human beings. I've always leaned toward the "both/and" mindset. It's a better way to understand, communicate, and make progress.

As a result, my brain naturally organizes ideas into quadrants. Sometimes, the best way to explain something is to sketch a simple visual or draw a line across a whiteboard.

Let me start with four core distinctions that have helped me across all disciplines:

1. Simple Concept

These are the basic truths we often overlook.
"Drink more water."
"Eat vegetables and fruit."
"Get good sleep."
"Walk more."

That's it. Simple—and effective. Like when you get lost in a small town and someone just points down the road and says, "That way." Simple isn't stupid. Simple works.

2. Complex Concept

Then there are things like space travel. I once read that the Voyager spacecraft passed Pluto within seconds of its projected arrival, decades after launch. That's not just rocket science—it's orbital mechanics, gravitational modeling, and predictive mathematics across time and space.

Human biology often falls into this category. The body's response to training, food, stress, and recovery is a complex process. Not unknowable, but intricate.

3. Simplified Instruction

One of my former throwers recently got hired as a coach. She asked for all the technical cues I'd used with her. I gave her a handful:

"Stretch."
"Spanky."
"1-2-3."
"3a-3b-3c."
She said, "That's it?"

Yep. Simple—but not easy. A few clear cues, rooted in deep understanding, can carry years of wisdom.

4. Complex Instruction

Then there are things that require a full checklist. Like flying a commercial airplane. When I glance into the cockpit before a flight and see pilots going through those checklists, I breathe a little easier.

I can ride a bike, drive a car, and operate a pickup truck—but flying 300 people across the country? That demands training, repetition, and discipline. That's complex instruction for a complex task.

So now, the Art of Coaching Quadrant!

	Complex Concept	Simple Concept
Simplified Instruction	The Art of Teaching/Coaching	"Sure, Of Course!"
Complicated Instruction	"Sure, Of Course!"	*Bullshit*

We don't mind simple instructions for simple tasks. "Where's the bathroom?" "Down the hall." Perfect.

And we should respect complex instructions when complexity is justified. I'm not going to argue with a physicist about gravity.

But here's the problem…

When Bullsh*t Masquerades as Wisdom

Sorry, Gentle Reader, but sometimes the nonsense gets thick. Especially in fitness.

When I see an influencer take something as beautifully simple as "eat more fruit" and spin it into a blend of faux science, conspiracy theory, and pseudomedical jargon that ends with **"buy my supplements,"** I call it what it is:

Bullsh*t.

Yes, every field has its nonsense. But the fitness industry seems to have graduated from it, with honors.

Here's how you know you're with a master coach, teacher, or counselor:

They take something incredibly complex and make it feel simple.

That's the art of coaching.

One tiny cue. One small insight.

And suddenly, a tangled knot of complexity unravels into clarity.

That's the job. ***Make the complex simple***—without watering it down.

…and The Curse of Michael Scott

I never watched the American version of *The Office* during its original run. Like many people, my life alternates between periods of seeming insanity and long stretches of quiet. When *The Office* first aired, I was working two full-time jobs—professor and teacher (and coach!)—while also handling countless pickups and drop-offs during that hectic phase of parenting.

Later, I bought the complete series and fell in love with the early seasons and the antics of the Dunder Mifflin crew.

Michael Scott, played brilliantly by Steve Carell, not only managed the office but also dabbled in improv (comedy without a script), screenwriting (his epic *Threat Level Midnight*), and a host of other hobbies. He considered himself an expert in many fields, and even included an exercise montage in his film.

Part of the comedic genius of the Scott character was his unwavering confidence in whatever field he dabbled in—including his infamous parkour introduction, a chaotic tribute to the stunt-heavy opening of the Daniel Craig *James Bond* reboot, *Casino Royale*. Hopefully, the stuntmen survived…on both shows.

Around the same time I was watching *The Office*, I discovered two researchers and a concept that helped me understand many of the frustrations I've had with the fitness industry. It's called the **Dunning-Kruger Effect**:

"Coined in 1999 by then-Cornell psychologists David Dunning and Justin Kruger, the eponymous Dunning-Kruger Effect is a cognitive bias whereby people who are incompetent at something are unable to recognize their own incompetence. And not only do they fail to recognize their incompetence, they're also likely to feel confident that they actually are competent."

—https://lsa.umich.edu/psych/news-events/all-news/faculty-news/the-dunning-kruger-effect-shows-why-some-people-think-they-re-gr.html

It's often jokingly called "Mount Stupid." I'm sure every reader has met someone with just enough knowledge to be dangerous.

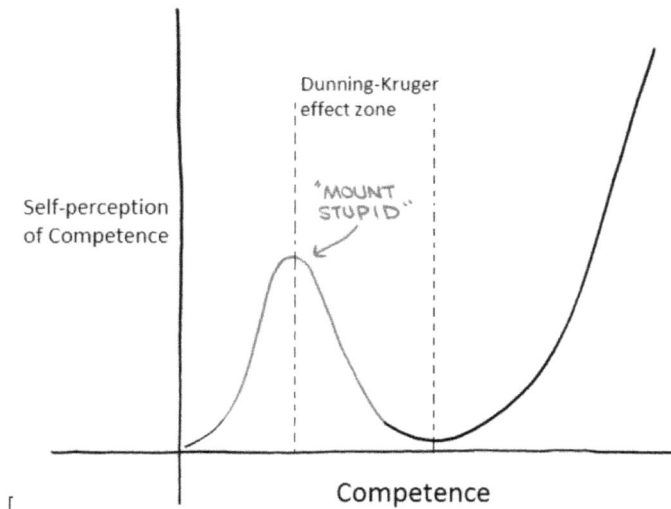

From: https://psychology.stackexchange.com/questions/17825/ what-is-the-primary-source-of-the-mount-stupid-graphic

In my case, I knew practically **everything** about weightlifting by the time I was fourteen. Honestly, I had some decent insights, and I even told Future Danny—my 64-year-old self fifty years in the future—to make sure to keep doing full-body lifts.

From the summit of Mount Stupid, I could see a future I thought I understood. Now, Future Danny looks back on decades of workshops, books, articles, discussions, certifications, and competitions—mountains of material that I had yet to climb.

Knowing a little seems like a LOT at first. I'm always reminded of an article I read from Reader's Digest where a nuclear warfare specialist was asked: "Wouldn't it be better if we just got rid of all the atomic weapons?"

The expert lowered his head and mumbled into the microphone: "If only it were that simple."

It's like telling a coach that we need to score more points: "If only it were that simple."

Oh… and the Michael Scott connection? With a sweep of the hand, one could say that he spends too much time on Mount Stupid. Everyone knows a blowhard who is always the expert…on everything.

And usually wrong.

And…that would make a great point. But…there's a different story I am not "proud" of, but it is funny.

Under the pressure of workshops, a microphone in hand and a crowd in front of me, I've accidentally called the Dunning-Kruger Effect the "Dunder Mifflin Effect" at least half a dozen times.

It makes me look like I spent a lot of time on Mount Stupid. But it is also always a funny moment.

Overcomplicating the basics of anything in any field is not a sign of sophistication; it often reveals a lack of understanding by the coach, trainer, or teacher.

Chapter Three

Health, Fitness, and the Art of Coaching: What Really Matters

I've long held to Phil Maffetone's definition of health: **"Health is the optimal interplay of the organs."** It's a powerful, grounded reminder that health isn't just the absence of disease or the number on a scale. It's a dynamic state—something that can always get a little better, something that we often don't appreciate until it's gone.

Health is evident in blood test results, in quiet longevity, and in the steady, uneventful passage of years without chronic pain or the need for medication. Tumors, high blood pressure, and fainting spells aren't health. And yet, in a world obsessed with external performance, we confuse the *appearance* of wellness with the real thing.

Most days, I try to remind myself to breathe deeply, smile, and enjoy a moment of good health. It's a gift. But that's not fitness.

Fitness Is Not Health

Fitness is simpler. It's the ability to perform a specific task. A thrower is fit for throwing. A jumper is fit for jumping. A sprinter is fit for sprinting. Fitness is context-dependent—it doesn't necessarily imply health.

I once knew a man who dove into the shallow end of a pool, drunk, and broke his neck. He can't walk today, but he fathered two sons. He is, technically, fit for the task of procreation, even though many people might not see him as "fit" in the traditional sense.

This distinction matters. Too often, we conflate health and fitness, leading to dangerous assumptions about our bodies, our training, and our longevity.

Health or Fitness? Know the Difference

Let's look at a few common phrases and decide whether they reflect **health** or **fitness**:

1. **"Live long, drop dead."** → *Health.*

   Longevity without chronic disease reflects optimal internal function, not task-specific capacity.

2. **Longevity is part of this.** → *Health.*

   Living longer isn't necessarily about being able to sprint or lift; it's about sustainable well-being.

3. **"Everyone is an athlete."** → *Fitness.*

   This phrase implies that every person has tasks they can train for, from parenting to Olympic lifting.

4. **"Fitness is what you achieve on the path to athletics."** → *Fitness.*

   Fitness is developed in the process of performing tasks, whether those are athletic, occupational, or everyday.

5. **"___ is the fittest person on Earth."** → *Fitness.*

   This is a competition title, based on physical performance, not health metrics.

Chapter Four

Clarity in the Carriage...A Personal Reflection on Goals

Like many former collegiate athletes, I've often wished for just one more year of university-level competition. Honestly, a single day would be enough. Ever since I graduated and exhausted my eligibility, I've quietly hoped for another chance.

Not long ago, the NCAA lost a court case, and those of us who used up eligibility at junior colleges suddenly discovered—cue *Glory Days* by Bruce Springsteen—we might be entitled to *two more years* of collegiate competition.

I reached out to the head coach at the university where I volunteer. At first, he thought I was joking. I wasn't. I also contacted my old university. The throws coach there thought it was a *splendid* idea.

So, I started putting the pieces together. I assessed my age, training, and recent efforts and realized: I could actually do this. I wouldn't live in the dorms, but I could still compete well enough to place in a lot of track and field meets.

But. There were other things to consider.

Right around then, my granddaughter Elowen turned six months old. My daughter Kelly was also expecting. And suddenly, something smacked me right between the eyes.

I'd been consciously dieting—mostly fasting (see *Easy Strength for Fat Loss*)—to bring my bodyweight down and improve my odds of seeing my grandchildren's recitals, proms, and weddings. I like being lighter. I like being healthier. I like coaching. I like my schedule and the variety of work I do with different organizations.

Yes, a two-year return to collegiate competition would make a great story. It might even become a movie. My name in lights. Brad Pitt could play me—*if* he got into great shape.

But to be a thrower again, I'd need to bulk up. Old injuries would come out of retirement, too. And as I often say, I know I can handle *one more* injury. I'm just not sure I have *one more recovery* left in me.

Young Danny loves the idea of competing again. Future Danny wants to dance at those weddings. Both options are good. Both are aligned with my values. But I can't do both.

This kind of dilemma—choosing between two good things—is what many of us face with our physical and financial goals. It's why, every January, we see people flail and fail with those things called *New Year's Resolutions*.

Before we go further, let's be clear: resolutions are usually a great idea. The most popular ones in recent years are:

- Save more money
- Eat healthier
- Exercise more
- Lose weight
- Spend more time with family
- Quit smoking
- Cut back on spending

Honestly, who would grab someone and shout: "Stop saving! Stop exercising! Eat more junk!"? These are all noble, worthwhile aspirations. And ironically, the most popular resolution?

No resolutions!

Years ago, I wrote in a men's magazine that a better resolution would be to weigh *just one pound less* by the next New Year's Day. One pound. That's it. 365 days (or 366 if it's a leap year).

Since a pound of fat equals roughly 3,500 calories, you'd need to cut just nine calories a day. That's skipping two olives in your martini. Or sleeping ten minutes longer—sleep burns about 50–70 calories an hour.

But readers online roasted me. It wasn't "hardcore" enough. Not convict/Spartan/warrior/Ninja enough. Still, I can't think of a better national goal than simply slowing down the march toward more body fat.

When I coach people on goal-setting, they often confuse goals with *resolutions*. Or, in the words of Mary Poppins, resolutions become "pie crust promises": easily made, easily broken.

So, before launching into any goal-setting, I teach two concepts that *sound* similar but are *very* different:

1. **Goal Hijacking**
2. **Values Conflict** (or "Values Collision")

Goal Hijacking

Goal hijacking is a term I wish I had invented. We used to summarize it like this:

"When you're up to your ass in alligators, it's too late to ask why you drained the swamp."

You've likely experienced it. Maybe you decided to get in shape and joined an "elite" gym that emphasized high intensity over sound technique. Next thing you know, you're recovering from back, shoulder, and knee surgeries.

I coached an athlete who could have placed at nationals—until he broke his ankle in a church basketball game. And every time I scroll social media and feel tempted to chase the latest five-second fitness fad—ignoring my coach's advice—I'm flirting with hijacking my goals.

At a *Perform Better* event in Long Beach, I visited a famous used bookstore and discovered an entire aisle dedicated to diet books. That's when I realized you can predict the next big trend by simply observing what *was once popular*. Low-this and high-that in cycles. If it's high-protein this year, trust me, low-protein is coming.

Most people I know are on a high-carb breakfast, high-fat lunch, and a high-everything dinner with some alcohol to finish. Diet fads are classic goal hijackers. As I've said before:

"It worked so well, I stopped doing it."

These days, I'm tracking calories, walking 10,000 steps daily, sleeping well, and lifting three days a week. If you've read *The Armor Building Formula* or *Easy Strength for Fat Loss*, you know what I'm doing.

And somehow, I've stuck with it. At a recent workshop, someone asked about my changes in body composition. I told them I've lost **one pound a month for four years**.

Why the consistency? Because I have a crystal-clear long-term goal: dancing at my granddaughter's wedding. She's brand new, but I'm thinking decades ahead.

Recently, I tied my lifetime best in pull-ups: 14 reps. Same number I hit in 1974 at 162 pounds. When a friend asked, "What's your new goal?" I said:

"Fourteen."

That's all I wanted. Now I'm adding load for my chin-ups, carefully avoiding Middle-Aged Pull-Up Syndrome (MAPS...those cranky elbows).

Stay in the carriage. Keep your head inside. Stay the course.

I'm finally listening to my coach. And that makes me laugh, because *coach* means a carriage that takes you from here to there. Most of my coaching these days is just slapping people back *into* the carriage and keeping them focused on the "there."

Stay in the carriage. Keep your head inside. Stay the course.

What keeps you focused might just be a goal that brings you to tears. (More on that soon.)

Values Conflict

This concept comes from Patrick Ides. I alluded to it earlier when I talked about reliving my *Glory Days* and returning to collegiate throwing. That idea still inspires me.

However, doing that means gaining weight, lifting heavy, and waking up those old injuries.

Bang! Right into my deeper goal—living long and well enough to celebrate life's big events with my grandkids.

Both goals are great. Both inspire me. But they collided. And I had to choose.

High school seniors know this feeling. After years of being told where to go and what to do, suddenly they're handed thousands of career options, college choices, and life decisions. It's overwhelming.

Choosing a college is a values decision. I chose Utah State to throw the discus and to finally "grow up." But picking one school meant saying no to hundreds of others.

I've seen it in kids and grandkids. Go to the toy store and say, "Pick ONE." They squirm.

As for me? There are two images that bring tears to my eyes. Go ahead and call me a snowflake—some guy on a forum has already done so. But he didn't leave a name or address, so here goes:

1. **Dancing at my grandkids' weddings.** I want to be there.
2. **My daughter saying, "Look, Dad, there's Bingo on Wednesday and pudding. You like pudding!"**

That second one? That's being put in "the home." To quote Harry Nilsson, "I'd rather be dead than wet the bed."

Those two visions keep me walking my 10,000 steps. They help me say no to sweets, seconds, and "another round." They give me clarity.

And clarity—especially about what you *don't* want—is what keeps you in the carriage on the way to *there*.

Chapter Five

What Do You *Really* Want? Training with Purpose, Tools, and Truth

Part of my job is asking people a deceptively simple question:

"What do you want?"

Now, I'm not a department-store Santa. I'm a strength coach. I don't have a magic sack full of six-packs, dream glutes, and unlimited energy. What I *do* have is a small collection of tools—proven, effective, and simple. But none of them matter until we answer that question honestly.

What We Want... Isn't Always What We Need

Most answers to "What do you want?" are predictable:

- *"I want to get leaner and have abs like I see on TV."*
- *"I want to look better and feel better. I want more energy."*
- *"I want to look like I did at age [fill in the blank]."*
- *"I want a pony."*

(Spoiler: I always want a pony. It might be the most realistic goal on that list.)

But here's the rub: **what we want isn't the real answer. What we *need* is.**

The best coaches help people discover and pursue what they *need*, not just chase surface-level desires.

Who Needs to Focus on "Needs"?

So, who should focus on **needs** over **wants**?

Most People I Know

These are everyday adults juggling work, family, stress, and the challenges of aging. They often *want* to look like their 20-year-old selves but *need* sleep, strength, movement, and recovery.

Collison Occupations and Elite Athletes

Tactical and high-level athletes *seek* high performance, but what they *truly need* is longevity, joint health, and foundational support to maintain optimal performance. This is the toughest blend of qualities… elite performance blended with longevity is a difficult recipe.

Any and all Active Athletes.

Even weekend warriors or recreational competitors benefit from a "needs-first" lens: smarter programming, fewer injuries, and longer careers.

To help you start looking at needs, we need to flex our mental might and look at some tools.

Time, Treasure, and Talents: The First Toolbox

In church work, there's a familiar call for support: time, treasure, and talents. These three pillars sustain the mission and also serve as a powerful lens for evaluating nearly everything in the world of fitness, including equipment, exercise selection, and programming decisions.

Let's break it down.

Time

This one seems obvious, but time is a slippery concept in health, fitness, longevity, and performance.

A high school senior at the end of a sports season doesn't have much time left, but also has *a lifetime* ahead to shape their future. Learning a skill or discipline that takes decades is a beautiful, slow journey… *if* you have the time to invest.

Boxing and strength coach Steve Baccardi once made a brilliant decision:

"If an exercise takes more than 15 minutes to teach the majority of my athletes, I cut it."

It's a harsh filter, but practical. Olympic lifts took me *years* to master. But they paid off big in my discus career. That was time well spent.

Time, as Einstein reminded us, is relative. And in fitness, it's everything.

Treasure

This usually feels straightforward—until it comes to buying equipment.

I once worked at a school that received a generous donation of five weight machines. The original cost (decades ago) was over $100,000.

And they were *completely useless*. Multiple adjustments, a short range of motion, and the ability to use the equipment by only one athlete at a time were just some of the problems.

Another time, a major equipment company offered me seven machines at a huge discount. Still, the cost of those seven items was equal to *two full weight rooms* we had built previously.

Yes, economics and cost-to-benefit analysis should be common sense, but those shiny machines can be tempting.

The truth? Sometimes the best tool is a loaded backpack and a hill. Spend wisely.

Talents

This one hits close to home.

I believe every coach, trainer, and teacher should be constantly upgrading their skill set. Not in a frantic, faddish way—but with consistent learning and refinement.

I once attended a national conference with a coach who was adamantly against the Olympic lifts. So, I asked:

"Can you do or coach the Olympic lifts?"

"No," she said. "I don't know them at all."

That answer still bothers me.

Your talents are your tools. If you don't sharpen them, don't be surprised when they fail you—or your athletes. Stay humble, stay curious, and keep learning.

One way to internalize this Time–Treasure–Talent model is to apply it to **recovery tools**.

Take the following list of recovery methods and ask yourself:

- **Time**: How long does it take to implement?

- **Treasure**: What does it cost in money and resources?

- **Talents**: Does it require special expertise or training?

Here's a quick contrast:

- **Sleep** takes 8–9 hours, sure—but it's *free* and universally effective.

- **Hot tubs** sound great—but outfitting your entire varsity football team with one each? Not so practical.

This framework isn't just for budgeting and logistics—it's a mindset that drives effective decision-making. Whether you're evaluating a new training tool, hiring staff, or planning a program, ask yourself:

What's the time commitment?

What's the real cost?

What skill or understanding does this demand?

Time, Treasure, and Talents—an old idea worth keeping in your modern coaching toolbox. In workshops, I have you mark up this list with the "Three Ts" and assess these three questions. The fun part of recovery tools is that someone always asks to add more and more "things" to the list.

Recovery Tools:	Time	Treasure	Talents
Sauna			
Hot Tub			
Massage			
Massage Gun			
Self-Massage			
Foam Roller			
Stretching			
Cryotherapy			
Ice Baths			
Cold Water Immersion			
Compression Garments			
Swimming			
Needling			
Original Strength			
Walking			
Yoga and associated forms of mobility work			
Rest/Naps			
Sleep			
Proper Nutrition			
Water (Drinking!)			
Contrast Baths			
Lacrosse/golf balls (Rolling on hot spots)			
Cupping			
Red light therapy			
Sauna blankets			
Lavender, mint, and the whole scent family			
Grounding or acupressure mats			
Ice packs			

We can also have some fun with foods. I know a lot of nutritionists hate the term "Superfoods," maybe there is too much Kryptonite in them, but I love the lists. I use the following lists for the Time, Treasure, and Talent assignment. Frankly, some people can't afford some of these items. In other cases, some may not be able to find these items in a local store or field, and there is also the issue of cooking and preparing them. Review these lists to see if you can identify your Superfoods.

Highlighted items are foods appearing in more than one list.

Men's Journal	Least Allergenic Dr. Elson Haas	Best Polyphenol Brad Pilon	Super Foods Good Housekeeping	For the Win Always mentioned
Almonds	Apricots	Black Currants	Avocados	Coffee
Beef	Beets	Blackberries	Beans	Olives
Coffee	Broccoli	Blueberries	Berries	Salmon
Eggs	Cabbage	Cherries	Broccoli	Water
Olive Oil	Carrots	Cloves	Citrus Fruits	
Salmon	Cauliflower	Dark Chocolate	Coffee	
Water	Cranberries	Dark Coffee	Dark Chocolate	
Yogurt	Halibut	Hazelnuts	Dark Leafy Greens	
	Herbal Teas	Olives	Fatty Fish	
	Honey	Orange Juice	Green Tea	
	Kale	Pecans	Olive Oil	
	Lamb	Plums	Turmeric	
	Olive Oil	Red Wine	Walnuts	
	Olives		Whole Grains	
	Pears			
	Rabbit			
	Rice			
	Salmon			
	Sole			
	Sweet Potatoes			
	Tapioca			
	Trout			
	Turkey			

Barbells and Beyond: Why Your Tools Matter

Let's take time, treasure, and talent into the weight room. Obviously, this isn't an exhaustive list, but I will share my inner dialogue with equipment.

I love barbells. I've used them since 1965, and I still believe they form the backbone of any effective strength program.

If all we ever did were military press and deadlift, we'd probably cover 80% of our needs. And when it's time to load heavy, barbells are unmatched. You can fine-tune from 55 to 60 pounds or load it to 700.

But barbells aren't everything. Here's why you should have these other tools in your coaching arsenal:

1. Kettlebells

Compact, versatile, and perfect for swings, get-ups, goblet squats, and more. Great for building power, grip, and mobility with ballistic and grind patterns.

2. Suspension Trainers (Straps)

Allow for scalable bodyweight work—such as rows, presses, and mobility drills—anywhere. Great for shoulder health and core integration.

3. Ab Wheel

Deceptively brutal. Few tools light up the anterior core and teach bracing like this. Easy to store. Easy to hate. Highly effective.

4. Dumbbells

Unilateral options, varied grip, and wide movement library. They're a staple for hypertrophy, rehab, and general strength.

5. Mini-Bands

Cheap, portable, and perfect for activating glutes, shoulders, and core. Ideal for warm-ups, rehab, and movement prep.

I always list these five in the Time, Treasure, and Talent conversation. Obviously, there are a host of tools, but these are the starting point (and, for me, there isn't much else I trust).

It's about meeting people where they are.

Each tool has its place. It's not about having everything—it's about knowing **why** you're using it.

Some Thoughts

Training isn't about magic formulas or secret programs. It's about meeting people where they are—asking them what they *want*, helping them discover what they *need*, and guiding them toward lasting progress.

Whether you're using a barbell or a mini-band, whether you're a busy grandparent or a SWAT officer, the principles stay the same:

- Know what you need.
- Choose the right tools.
- Train movements that last.

And always—always—keep asking the right questions. Let's shift to the key questions.

Chapter Six

The Big Three Questions

In the past, I introduced ten questions to help people gain clarity. But after a dozen or so workshops on the material, I realized that everything distilled down to just three:

- What's your goal?

- Will this goal expand your life for the better in most ways?

- How old are you?

What's Your Goal?

Goals tend to settle into two big heaps.

The first kind used to be more common—we'll call these **Scoreboard Goals**. These are the numbers we chase: a target body weight, weekend sales totals, and money raised for a school project. In individual sports like track and field, swimming, or Olympic lifting, athletes can aim for specific numbers to hit in a season or over a career.

Team sports are trickier, but most coaches would agree: beating a rival and winning a championship are top goals. Behind those? Dozens of smaller, often forgotten objectives that stack up toward a trophy.

Recently, **Process Goals** have gained popularity. Influenced by the work of BJ Fogg and the "Tiny Habits" movement, many of us are now trying to slowly turn the wheel toward progress. When I was asked recently how I changed my body composition, I said:

"I lost a pound a month for four years."

Cutting 100 calories a day and walking 10,000 steps won't yield instant change, but the habits—the process—add up. With process goals, you often need to learn a new skill, acquire tools or coaching, and—most of all—stick to the plan.

When I decided to incorporate more fermented foods into my diet, I took a local fermentation class. That hands-on experience expanded my understanding of the gut biome's critical role. If you can't cook, it's going to be hard to control your calories.

I've noticed three patterns in how people frame their goals: **A–B**, **A–Z**, and **A–Not A**.

- **A–B Goals**: This is the most common. "I'm here. I want to get there." I prefer short timelines for these—rarely more than six weeks.

- **A–Z Goals**: This happens when someone wants to look like they did 40 years ago, after decades of beer, pizza, and sweets— and they give me a four-week deadline. I'm all for massive transformations, but we need to break it down first.

- **A–Not A Goals**: Steve Ledbetter taught me this one. It's simple and often heartbreaking: "You see me? This? This is NOT me." Sometimes life just hits hard. Years of stress or neglect can make you feel like a stranger in your own body.

Strangely, both elite athletes and everyday people transition between all three at different points in their lives.

Will This Goal Expand Your Life?

This second question may be even more important than the first.

I've found myself quoting Peggy Lee's famous line a few too many times after watching someone work endlessly to reach a goal... and then reach it:

Is that all there is?
Is that all there is?
If that's all there is, my friends,
Then let's keep dancing.
Let's break out the booze and have a ball...
If that's all there is.
—Peggy Lee

I've achieved most of my goals: athletic scholarships, elite performance, fatherhood, financial security (I just hit a 40-year milestone in one area of my financial goals), and world travel. I love all of it.

But, as a friend said after waiting over two hours to see the *Mona Lisa*, "Is that all there is?"

As a coach, parent, and athlete, I try to set goals that **expand**. A few years ago, I watched a rabbi on TV give the best advice I've ever heard for mental, physical, and spiritual health—and for goal achievement.

He was asked about unhappiness. His response was simple:

"Examine your prepositions."

Prepositions, as we're told, are all the things a rabbit can do with a log: around it, above it, behind it, through it, and so on.

Now think of your goals. Who is *behind* you, encouraging you? Who is *around* you, supporting you? Who is *ahead* of you, showing the way?

I belong to several Intentional Communities. Five days a week, a group of us meet to train. I provide the space and knowledge; they bring enthusiasm and good cheer.

I also belong to a financial Intentional Community. We meet weekly to discuss progress, our vision of the future, and our relationship with money. It's easier to save and eliminate debt when you walk that path with someone.

How Old Are You?

I often joke: a year from now, this will be different.

If you're in your twenties, high school (hopefully) is in the rearview mirror. Maybe it's time to stop chasing high school goals. If you're over 22, a professional athletic career might be out of reach.

But!

You can still learn new sports and participate in competitions. You can master musical instruments, pick up new languages, and take to the stage. My favorite book, *The Sword in the Stone*, says it better than I ever could:

"The best thing for being sad," replied **Merlyn**, beginning to puff and blow, "is to learn something. That's the only thing that never fails. You may grow old and trembling in your anatomies, you may lie awake at night listening to the disorder of your veins, you may miss your only love, you may see the world about you devastated by evil lunatics, or know your honour trampled in the sewers of baser minds. There is only one thing for it then — to learn. Learn why the world wags and what wags it. That is the only thing which the mind can never exhaust, never alienate, never be tortured by, never fear or distrust, and never dream of regretting. Learning is the only thing for you. Look what a lot of things there are to learn." — T. H. White, *The Sword in the Stone*

I consider those the most beautiful words ever written about the ongoing value of education.

Check Feasibility

Before diving headfirst into a new goal, take a moment to check its feasibility. My usual checklist includes:

- Your DNA (genetics)
- Your family/social life
- Your personality
- Your geography

Being over seven feet tall is beneficial if you aspire to play in the NBA. Having newborn triplets can significantly impact your sleep schedule. Some personality types don't mesh well with certain sports. And if you want to dominate in ice hockey, it helps to live in Canada, not at the equator.

You can absolutely ignore this advice, but aligning your goals with your reality makes the path much easier.

When "Seeking" a Goal, Will Attaining It Make You Successful?

There's a well-worn cliché I think deserves more attention:

"People may spend their whole lives climbing the ladder of success, only to find, once they reach the top, that the ladder is leaning against the wrong wall."

Sometimes it's phrased another way:

"It's no fun to reach the top of the ladder only to discover it's propped against the wrong wall."

Or as the great San Franciscan Herb Caen once wrote:

"It is a funny thing—you work all your life toward a certain goal, and then somebody moves the posts on you."

You get the point.

I've known many people from my athletic career who achieved great goals, but were absolute disasters in life. I won't name names, but the "failed former superstar" is itself a cliché, not just in sports, but in the arts, business, and politics, too.

Now, to be clear: I'm all for goals. But achieving **a** goal isn't always the same as achieving **success**.

Earl Nightingale often said:

"Success is the progressive realization of a worthy goal or ideal."

So, yes—goal setting and success are intertwined. But as Nightingale emphasized, it must be a **worthy** goal.

> **But achieving a goal isn't always the same as achieving success.**

Nightingale went on to say that the most successful people in life are often schoolteachers and parents—those who dedicate themselves to building a better future.

Success is *progressive*. It's not just the destination—it's the journey. It's the process. I never quite reached my long-term goals as a discus thrower, but I can tell you exactly how close I came to achieving them. I can also tell you how much that pursuit shaped me, challenged me, and moved me forward in ways that matter far beyond numbers on a scoreboard.

Chapter Seven

Moving Ahead: The Model of The Art of Coaching

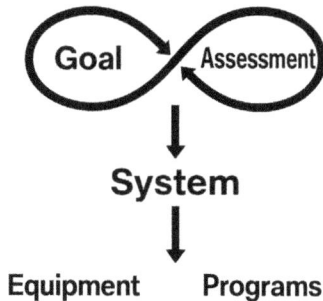

Moving Ahead: The Model of The Art of Coaching Graph

I've heard enough goal-setting lectures to know the old sailing cliché by heart: achieving a goal is like steering a sailboat into the wind. You may feel like you're moving away from your destination, but each tack—each course correction—brings you a little closer to your trusted harbor.

That's why **constant assessment** is so vital. I can't emphasize this enough: we need ongoing feedback, moment by moment, to guide progress.

As I often say, being a throws coach—or a strength coach—is, in many ways, a gift. When a thrower throws farther or a lifter lifts more, it's pretty clear: we're doing something right. But life isn't linear. And neither is progress. Regression and stagnation can mask deep improvements. Oddly, short-term gains can sometimes uncover long-term issues.

I've told this story many times:

When I was eighteen, my coach, Dick Notmeyer, left to attend the Montreal Olympics. During that stretch, I trained in the city at the Sports Palace. My dad drove me there—mostly to cover the ten-dollar day fee—and I started training.

That's why assessment must be ongoing.

My clean and jerks felt good. My personal best, walking in the door, was 270 pounds. But, thanks to kilos, the next logical jump was 271—and I made it.

My dad said it looked easy.
So I tried 282.
Then 292.
Then Dan Curiel walked in and said, "Try 137.5 kilos. You can make it." That's 303 pounds.

And I made it. I had shattered a milestone, breaking the 300-pound barrier and adding 33 pounds to my personal record—in about half an hour.

The problem?
I thought that was my new normal.
I figured the 400-pound lift was only a few good workouts away.

Reality, of course, crept in. Progress is rarely that fast. Often, it's glacial.

That's why **assessment must be ongoing**. Whether your goal is to reach port safely or simply get your bodyweight to stay down, the path is rarely direct. Sometimes the goal feels further away than it should. At other times, it seems closer than it actually is. Without regular check-ins and honest feedback, your target will continue to drift.

Assessment allows for tiny adjustments that keep us on track—even when we need to adapt, learn, and grow. It's not just about setting a goal. It's about steering. Coaching, like sailing, is not just an art. It's the art of adjustment.

Systems Support the Goals and Assessments

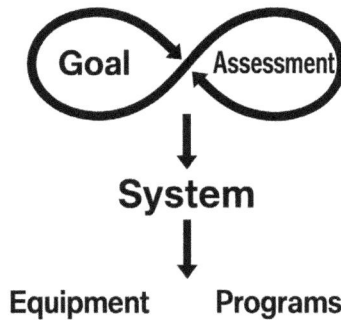

I've used a simple definition for the word *system* for a long time:
A system is a set of parts combined into a whole.

As an American football coach, systems allow us to condense a mountain of information into just a few words. Consider these:

- Right Two, 23

- Split, 14

- Cowboy 4

They're all describing the same play: a basic dive to the right by the running back, just delivered through three different systems.

I often emphasize **systems over habits** when talking about life changes. Saying "I will floss my teeth every morning" is fine. But the **system** I use is to buy bags of floss sticks, stash them in every bathroom, and keep a full supply in the driver's side cubby. When I drive, I floss.

Nice statements are nice. **Systems get things done.**

I have three rules for systems in fitness and sport that help keep me sane:

Rule One: Improve with Subtraction

Most people have experienced this at a party or a family gathering: someone leaves, and the event gets better. We all know that one person who sucks the oxygen out of a room. When they walk out the front door early, the whole place lifts.

Every gym I've ever worked in improved when we cleaned out the junk. Dust, spiderwebs, outdated machines—gone. We didn't even need to fill the space; just leaving it empty felt like a win.

I often revisit my exercise selection system—the *movement matrix*—and always find it improves when I remove clutter. When I added the hip thrust to the hinge category, it allowed me to eliminate several complex, hard-to-teach movements.

Systems get better with less, not more.

Rule Two: New Components Must Improve the Whole

This rule might seem obvious. You might even ask, "Why do we even need to say this?" But trust me: we do.

It comes down to the word that clarifies everything from body composition to financial security:

Enough.

What's *enough* body fat? What's *enough* monthly income?

Too often, we add things—tools, exercises, toys—without asking if they're actually making the system better. When I meet with exercise equipment salespeople, I always ask:

"What does this do better?"

Usually, I get a vague hand wave and a claim that the *Magic Muscle Machine 5000* can do all sorts of things— "just as well as…" whatever I already have. So, why replace a barbell that has served the world for over a century with a machine the size of a truck?

However, when I adopted kettlebells, I discovered that the modern swing did more than my current tools. I dismissed suspension trainers at first—until I tried single-arm planked rows. Those tools improved my system and allowed me to eliminate exercises that no longer served me.

Rule Three: A System Survives the Founder

As I write this, Coach Ralph Maughan has been gone for over two decades. Yet you can still see his influence in the technique of today's top discus throwers.

Meanwhile, if you flip through old muscle magazines, you'll see miracle machines and training systems that vanished along with the dodo.

In every sport, you'll find offensive and defensive systems that outlived their creators. That's the power of a system: it grows, adapts, and evolves long after the founder is gone.

And that, truly, is the **secret of long-term success**.

My System

- Movement—appropriate and fundamental—is primary.

- Strength must be in a relationship with the Goal. (Load is easy to increase but must be appropriate.)
- *Little and Often over the Long Haul.*

There's a common critique I hear:

"That's not a system. That's just a list of principles!"

Fair enough. But systems, at their core, are built around something deeper:

My system is based on constant vigilance toward the GOAL.

Because...

**The goal
is to keep
the goal
the goal.**

I've been using that phrase since 1996. It originated from a conversation about an organization that had strayed from its mission. I said, "The mission is to keep the mission the mission."

It was oddly profound. In coaching—and in life—it became obvious:

Coaching is about keeping the goal achiever in the four-wheeled vehicle that gets them from *here* to *there*.

That vehicle?

It's called a **coach**.

And please—call me *Coach*.

Chapter Eight

Equipment and Programs

When it comes to equipment, these are simply the **tools we use**. I've trained for Olympic lifting meets using nothing more than broomsticks and hills. That's what I had. I didn't have a lovely, air-conditioned room with platforms, bumper plates, barbells, chalk, and all the trimmings.

And you know what? Sometimes, **not** having the perfect setup makes you think, and thinking is often underappreciated.

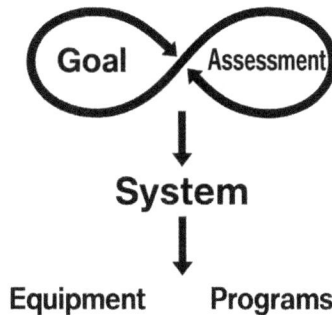

I've always embraced the challenge of training without optimal facilities. I once coached national champions in the discus without a throwing ring or even a field. We improvised, and in many ways, it made things better.

My home gym is brutally hot in the summer and freezing in the winter. The training adapts with the seasons, and my body thrives on that adaptation.

So yes, equipment is simply the "stuff" you use. Examples?

- Bodyweight

- Grass, sand, ground

- Bells (of any kind)

- Rocks

- Machines

- Complex tech

- Anything!

It makes sense to regularly assess your time, treasure, and talent—and to review every piece of equipment you currently use or are considering. Are your tools serving the mission?

Programs tend to follow equipment.

Through the years, I've fielded plenty of interesting questions:

- "Can I do an Olympic lifting program with only kettlebells?"

- "Can I follow a barbell-based plan using only bodyweight?"

I'm still working on the best answers to those questions.

At the core, programming comes down to three simple points:

1. **Do no harm.**

2. **The goal is to keep the goal the goal.**

3. **The path: Someone has probably done it before. Follow them.**

Let's take them one at a time.

1. Do No Harm

Hippocrates gave us the first key to coaching or leading anyone on a meaningful path:

Primum non nocere.
First, do no harm.

That's the better-known of his two principles. The other? *Do good.* And while "do good" sounds simple, it must be measured somehow. For strength or throws coaches, that part is relatively easy: more weight on the bar or more distance on the implement.

Here's the quote:

"The physician must ... have two special objects in view with regard to disease, namely, to do good or to do no harm."

And as simple as it sounds, I've seen it violated in disastrous ways.

A hammer thrower's career ended by a jumping drill.

A high jumper's career was ruined by a church league basketball game.

Countless "moronic" drills that merely exhaust the athlete and accomplish nothing on the field of play.

Just like with systems, programming often improves with **subtraction**.

Please memorize this:

Just because you can, doesn't mean you should.

Avoid silly gym contests. Avoid trending nonsense. Avoid saying:

"Hold my beer and watch this."

Get rid of the crap. Get rid of the excessive "conditioning." And above all, **focus on the goal.**

2. The Goal is to Keep the Goal the Goal

This is the heart of every frustrated coach, administrator, teacher, parent, and athlete. The *Urban Dictionary* explains it perfectly:

"So overcome or preoccupied by various tangential worries, problems, or tasks that one loses sight of the ultimate goal or objective." (The explanation of the quote: 'When you are up to your neck in alligators, it's easy to forget that the goal was to drain the swamp.')

I spend a lot of time helping young coaches trim the fat from their programs. Here's my summary:

- Throwers throw.
- Jumpers jump.
- Sprinters sprint.
- Runners run.

That was my job as a head track and field coach. But I still go to practices and see throwers sprinting and jumping and doing all kinds of things… except throwing.

Yes, they might be in decent "shape," but they're not doing something crucial.

They're not throwing.

Let me make this clear:

> My throwers throw.
> A lot.
> Every practice.

That's it. That's the job.
The goal is to throw far.
My job is to keep the goal the goal

3. Follow the Path

The final point is oddly simple:

Find someone who's done what you want to do. Do what they did.

I really want to stop right there:

Do what they did.

My discus hero, Glenn Passey, spent his summers on a dairy farm doing farmer walks and tossing hay bales into barn rafters. In the fall, he Olympic lifted—working toward bodyweight numbers on the clean and press and the snatch—and, of course, threw a lot.

He followed Coach Maughan's advice exactly: "Lift weights three days a week, throw the discus four days a week—for the next eight years."

When I did what Passey and Maughan told me to do…
I got pretty good.

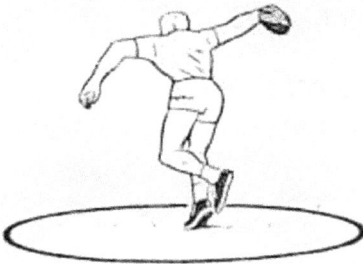

Coach Maughan's drawing of Glenn Passey for an article in 1963.

Chapter Nine

Stay on the Right Path: Three Principles of Coaching

I follow three basic coaching principles to help me stay on the right path. They're simple, interconnected, and, to some, probably obvious:

- The Prisoner's Dilemma
- Little and Often Over the Long Haul
- Concept–Drill–Frankenstein's Monster

The Prisoner's Dilemma

I've used this challenge with coaches and trainers for years, and now I'll pose it to you:

If, for whatever reason, you were allowed only three fifteen-minute sessions a week, what would you do?

Don't worry about *why* you're limited—pretend you're a political prisoner or something. What would you do in those three short workouts to reach your goal?

Whatever your answer is…
That should be the core of your training.

As a discus thrower, I'd perform full turns into a wall using a powerball, and then snatch or front squat every ten throws. That would be my entire plan. Because that *is* the plan.

Josh Hillis had a brilliant answer for fat loss:

"I'd do food preparation!"

This question reveals what **you** believe is essential—the non-negotiables. Once you've identified that, your job as a coach is to make sure the athlete actually *does* it.

And sometimes, the answers are surprising. A baseball coach once told me he wouldn't include much batting practice—because hitting, in his view, didn't always improve with reps. That's a bold answer. But it was honest.

Ask the question. Let the answer become the core of your future programming.

Little and Often Over the Long Haul

I first heard this phrase, "Little and Often Over the Long Haul, from Coach Ralph Maughan, though the idea has been echoed by many. I was sitting in his office, and he had just summed discus throw training with this point I love to review:

**Consistently.
Repeatedly.
Relentlessly.**

"If you want to be good at the discus, lift weights three days a week and throw four days a week... for the next eight years."

Most people miss that last part—**for the next eight years.**

There's no two-week transformation program for mastery. If you want to be great, you must get out to that prison courtyard and train. Consistently. Repeatedly. Relentlessly.

There are no overnight sensations in mastery. There is only commitment over time.

Concept – Drill – Frankenstein's Monster

This final principle helps us avoid a common trap in coaching: **mastering the minors**.

When I teach a movement, I begin with the **concept**—the big picture. If someone understands the concept, I don't worry much about breaking it down. They're ready.

For example:

The concept of the squat is to drop between the legs, not on top of them. If the athlete naturally falls between the thighs, they've got it. No drills needed. Congrats.

But when something's missing or awkward, that's when we go to **drills**. Sometimes, yes, *the drill is the skill*, but drills should never cloud the larger picture. They are tools to reinforce the concept, not replace it.

And now we come to the **Frankenstein problem**.

Frankenstein's monster was a collection of mismatched parts. Too many coaches approach training the same way:

- "This is your ankle."

- "This is your knee."

- "This is your hip."

Ignore the parts as long as you can. Let the body—and the mind—figure things out. Motor learning thrives on holistic repetition. Only after completing numerous reps with clear limits should you begin to examine the weak link, joint by joint or cue by cue.

Bringing It All Together

Combine these three principles:

1. **Decide what really matters.** Ask the prisoner's dilemma and make that answer the core.

2. **Give it time.** A lot of time. Lay out the months and years needed to get there.

3. **Zoom out.** Teach the whole before the parts. Don't let drills or detail override understanding.

Now that we know the client's goal and where they are in life, it's time to develop the qualities they need to reach point B.

And at the end of the day, it all comes back to assessment.

As we say in the gym:

If you ain't assessing, you're guessing.

Chapter Ten

Assessing These Rules

Most people have experienced the magic of **addition by subtraction**. At a party or in the workplace, when someone leaves, everything suddenly feels better. In my coaching career, eliminating traditional conditioning methods (especially dreadful things like wind sprints) lifted the mood and energy of entire training sessions.

Subtraction is often easy to assess. You feel like you've gained time, space, clarity, and everything just works better.

Rule Two—that new components must improve the overall organism—is more difficult to assess. When you add something (a new drill, exercise, tool, supplement, job, or relationship), how do you know it's working?

For this, I use a mental model called **The Two Test Tubes**.

In one test tube, you place everything you invest in this new idea: time, money, attention, energy, and even goodwill (such as over-tipping or offering kindness).

In the other test tube, you place what you get back: results, feedback, memories, joy, clarity, or yes, even money.

Cost to Benefit Ratios

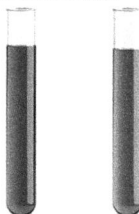

Now, imagine marking the second tube at about **20% full**. I use that as a benchmark. If what you're adding gives you back **at least** that much return, it may be worth keeping. If it's filling up to **80%**, you've struck gold.

Yes, this borrows from the **Pareto Principle**—the classic 80/20 rule. It's a business cliché, but still one of the best tools I know for judging results.

I say "yes" to a lot of new opportunities and ideas. I toss them into the test tubes and grade them like this:

- **A** — Like in school, this is the best you can do. You invest 20% of your effort and get 80% of the reward. When someone starts doing goblet squats and farmer walks, and it rekindles their love of training—that's an A. Royalties from old work fit here, too. Few things feel better than a check in the mail for something you did a decade ago.

- **B** — This is the fair trade. You put in your time and energy, and get roughly the same back. That's still a win.

- **C** — These are the minor exchanges. You give a little, get a little. Harmless, but don't expect them to change your life. I still try a lot of these, because some Cs eventually reveal themselves as hidden As.

- **F** — These are the energy vampires. You give and give and get almost nothing back. If something is draining you and offering no return, **stop**. Right now.

When you pick up a new idea from a workshop or article, assess it through this lens. If it takes months or years to master but only gives a tiny benefit—or worse, drags you backward—let it go. Learn, adjust, move on.

But if something is easy to implement and transforms your training or your life, celebrate it. Give it an A.

This simple framework helps me evaluate nearly everything—from training exercises to relationships to movies on airplanes.

A: Low Cost, High Return

These are the hidden gems.

Minimal time, effort, or investment—but a strangely huge benefit.

Examples:

- Walking
- Drinking water
- Protein
- Olympic lifts for throwers
- Lifetime royalties
- Longstanding friendships that lift you up

These are **the jewels of life**.

B: Reasonable Cost, Reliable Return

You get out what you put in. It's steady, dependable, and respectable.

Examples:

- Fiber (yes, I always start with fiber…what fiber you tend to put into your body, well, you tend to get it out)
- The 9–5 job
- Classic barbell lifts
- Marvel movies
- Writing regularly

These are what keep the lights on and the wheels turning. They're also how you create the *space* and *stability* to discover more As.

C: Low Entry Cost, Variable Return

C grades are small bets—little adventures, a new exercise, an unfamiliar idea, or a chance encounter. Most won't change your life, but some might. And occasionally, one of them becomes an A.

Sometimes they're just "good enough."

Examples:

- Trying hip thrusts for the first time (total game changer for me)
- Saying yes to a new business idea
- Watching *Nomadland* or *Past Lives* on a quiet night. Great movies, but I might only watch them once. I've seen *The Godfather* and *Galaxy Quest* dozens of times…
- Testing a new diet, lift, or recovery tool

C-grade ideas are how we *find* the As. And if they stay Cs? That's fine. We still learn.

F: High Cost, Little to No Return

Run away.

If something demands your time, energy, money, or emotional bandwidth—and gives you nothing back—it's an F.

Examples:

- Exercises that hurt and don't help
- One-way friendships that drain you

- Bad investments (financial or personal)
- Endless complaining phone calls from people who never ask about *your* day

If you notice that a relationship consistently drains you without ever refueling you… It may be time to consider a boundary.

In short:

Stop F-ing around and drop the Fs.

Cost to Benefit Ratios

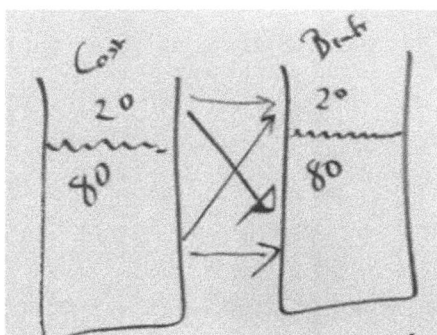

This is from one of my workshops where I drew this idea on a whiteboard. If the Cost is low and the Benefits are high, that's our A grade. If we see nice benefits from a reasonable cost, that's our Bs; Cs are the little experiments that might shift to As…Fs are those horrid things that take all your time, treasure, and talents and return little. The 80/20 principle here is based on Pareto's Law, and it's a fun way to connect the concepts.

The best advice I can give: **Grow the As**.

I've seen many C-grade ideas—tiny movements, strange cues, oddball workshops—suddenly bloom into life-changing A-grade staples. A good example? Hip thrusts. I tried them as a curiosity, and they stuck.

But you only find these by trying. You must stay curious. Say yes sometimes.

Try small. Fail fast. Learn always.
Grow the As.

When someone I trust—someone I love—tells me, "Try this," I do. Many of those small nudges have changed my life. Some were As in disguise.

Rule Three reminds us: great systems outlive their founders. A thriving, lasting system reflects not only the wisdom of the originator but the strength of those who carried the torch forward. Institutions that endure show their history in rings of growth, like a tree—visible, evolving, and deeply rooted.

Try small. Fail fast. Learn always.

This is true in every field.

There is one more question that we all need to answer before we begin the journey:

What's enough?

Enough!

I'm always amazed at some of the conversations I have.

I've talked with parents worried that their 13-year-old son will suddenly turn into Mr. Universe after signing up for a weightlifting class. He hasn't even picked up a single bell yet, and already we're stressing about him reaching the genetic ceiling of elite muscle development.

Let me be clear: it's not just a matter of waving around a few weights. Achieving a single-digit body fat percentage while maintaining elite-level muscle mass requires **years** of dedication, consistency, self-sacrifice, and unwavering focus.

And honestly, most people don't need to worry about looking like a prize-winning bodybuilder or a professional model. DNA plays a significant role, and so does the level of 24/7 commitment it takes to reach those extremes. It's not just effort—it's *life consumption*.

So the real question becomes:

What is "enough" for you?

If your goal is to look like a top-tier fitness competitor, there are better resources than what I offer. I would simply caution that the road to that level comes with a cost. In the words of *Rocky Balboa*:

"If you want to dance, you gotta pay the piper."

Each week, I attend an Intentional Community gathering focused on finances. It's modeled on my training philosophy: bring like-minded people together to share resources, energy, and wisdom. Whenever someone new joins our group, we always ask the same first question:

"What's enough for you?"

You *could* save or invest 50% of your income. You *could* use the public library for all your entertainment. You *could* shut off the heat and A/C, walk everywhere, and sell off every possession you own. You *could* do that.

I couldn't. But somebody else might—and that's great.

It's the same when people write to my podcast. Sometimes I'll say:

"For somebody else, that's a great idea or experiment to try.

For me? No, not so much."

Now let's bring that same question back to body composition:

What's "enough" for you?

Increasing lean body mass while maintaining reasonable body fat levels offers lifelong benefits. LBM—lean body mass—is one of the most powerful indicators of health and longevity. It supports your **health span**—the quality of your years, not just the quantity.

I've long believed in a long-term approach to strength and health. That principle has guided nearly every training and lifestyle decision I've made.

I'm deeply grateful to my younger self for lifting, walking, and staying (mostly) away from being too stupid. Maintaining a body fat level within a reasonable range goes a long way toward preventing the ravages of diabetes, cardiovascular disease, and other lifestyle-related ailments we'd rather avoid.

My programs—first and foremost—are systems that promote:

- Excellent health
- Improved performance
- Broad-spectrum fitness
- A longer, happier life

And that's **enough** for me.

Chapter Eleven

Teaching Coaching

The concept of enough opens the door to our next discussion. Nothing is going to challenge our Two Towers of Coaching (with a nod to J. R. R. Tolkien):

1. The need to understand the cost-to-benefit ratio of every training idea, tool, system, piece of equipment, and program.

2. The importance of being goal-focused.

I have hammered "The goal is to keep the goal the goal" for decades to my athletes and fellow coaches. It doesn't always get traction.

Honestly, I don't think I can bear to hear one more story about a team that was "in better shape" than the opponent… and still lost by a record number of points. No one adds points to the basketball scoreboard for smaller waistlines. No one checks how many push-ups a marathoner can do at the finish line. It's not about being in shape—it's about being in shape for the task at hand.

This is why **coaching needs both a system and a mindset**:

- Coaching needs a system.
- Coaching needs steps.
- Coaching needs to be flexible to change instantly.
- Coaching needs to have rigid standards.
- Coaching is teaching.
- Coaching is leading.
- Coaching is the art of blending *both/and* with *either/or*.

This blend is the art. The logic, structure, and tools of coaching are the science. So, how do we teach coaching?

Systemic and Systematic Education

My motto as an administrator was simple:

"Repetition is the mother of implementation."

So if I tend to repeat myself, consider it illuminating, not annoying.

I've always loved **systematic** approaches. It's the core of how we learn math: we begin with counting, move through arithmetic, and eventually land in the world of differential equations. Step by step, brick by brick. Many team sports follow the same path—years of layered instruction, repetition, and experience just to get to the intermediate level.

In disciplines like geometry or theology, a good system starts with **givens**—those assumptions or known truths we accept up front—and follows a logical process to reach the "to prove." In sports, those givens often include **genetics and geography**. Where you're born, what your body can do, and the resources you have access to all play a role, no matter how good your coaching is.

Systemic education is different. It's not linear—it's immersive. It's the way we typically learn religion, join the military, or fall in love with a sports team. You don't join the Marine Corps by filling out paperwork and watching training videos. You go to boot camp. You are dipped in the waters of the experience. It's learn-by-doing in its rawest, purest form.

But here's the caveat: immersion isn't always better.

Imagine this: your houseplants get aphids. You panic and throw ten different sprays, powders, and home remedies at them. A few days later, the aphids are dead—and so are the plants. What worked? What caused harm? What helped? You can't tell.

Training can be like this, too. Start a new program, overhaul your diet, take a cabinet full of supplements, and lose one pound over two months. Which of those variables helped? Likely, none.

There is a time and place for **systematic learning**—a checklist, a progression, a known path. But sometimes, the only way to find out if the water is cold… is to dive in.

Right or wrong, I've been diving into strength and conditioning since 1965. And yes, I've been wrong a lot.

As I review the ideas, drills, diets, and insights I've tried over the years, I can see the stories behind each one. Some led to breakthroughs. Some led to injuries, surgeries, and long rehabs. But the silver lining is this: you don't need to repeat every mistake I've made.

Still, I encourage you to make some mistakes. **Real lessons aren't often learned on a beach with a cocktail in hand.** As Oscar Wilde said:

"Experience is simply the name we give our mistakes."

And I've got plenty of experience.

I started work on The Art of Coaching years ago as a response to the lack of **systematic** education in strength training. Much of my coaching philosophy is a call to walk the path, step by step. Add the right things to the soil. Learn to do one thing well before layering complexity.

Steve Baccari, a boxing coach from Boston, gave us one of the clearest models I've ever heard:

"He severely limits the number of variables and tracks one while keeping the rest constant. Two groups of fighters of similar ability are doing the

same things—except for one—for a certain number of weeks. The proof of what works better comes out in the ring."—Pavel, Simple & Sinister

This is the coaching mindset at its best. Simple. Isolated. Measurable. Honest.

A Framework for Thinking About Coaching

Let's clarify two important contrasts that often arise in both education and coaching:

Systemic	Systematic
Immersive	Step-by-step
Culture	Checklist
"This is who we are."	"This is what we do."

In coaching—as in geometry—we begin with:

- **Given:** What you have (genetics, geography, resources)

- **To Prove:** The goal

The coach's job is to connect the two.

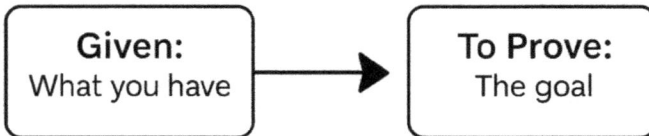

A great coaching toolkit draws on both *systemic* and *systematic* education. American football, in particular, has traditionally embraced both approaches. A typical season starts with training camp. When I was growing up, "two-a-days" were a staple of my childhood. We'd wake early, head to school, and essentially spend the entire day practicing. Two full practices a day. Putting on sweat-soaked pads for the afternoon session remains one of the grosser memories of my athletic life.

We learned the systems, formation by formation, play by play. Skills like blocking, tackling, and ball protection were drilled relentlessly. To this day, I can diagram plays like *the Left One, 37 Wedge Fly,* or *West Special,* along with the responsibilities of every player.

At the same time, we were immersed in the program's *culture.* Each practice reminded us that we were *earning* the right to wear the school colors and carry on the team's traditions. I've coached in programs where athletes touch a sign as they exit the locker room—some of those alumni return decades later to tap it again, with reverence.

Proper coaching bridges the immersive power of systemic education with the structure of systematic learning. I can speak on the phone with a former athlete, mention that my current thrower doesn't "keep Spanky," and immediately sense understanding on the other end. More often than not, that former athlete will share a story that helps the new thrower—and deepens our shared immersion.

In the discus, the movement pattern is "Stretch–1–2–3." But our *identity* includes phrases like:

- "Last throw, best throw."
- "Throw far or die."

That last one may sound extreme, but the athletes *insist* it stays. Why?

Because:

This is who we are.

Chapter Twelve

Shark Habits and Pirate Maps

It's time to share the two best TOOLS I know to keep the focus on the goals we all agreed on. To stay on task, we need to constantly clear the clutter. I preach and teach Shark Habits (make a decision and be done with it) and Pirate Maps (a small list of daily "to-dos" to keep you on the path to your big goal), and I don't know of a better system of achieving goals and dreams...by simply doing what is important!

Shark habits have a profound impact on mental health.

I live by my shark habits. If I open an email, I answer it. If I receive a wedding invitation, I respond and then go online to buy the gift. When I open my closet, I see 12 of the exact same black V-neck shirts, and I put one on.

It's simple: one bite and it's gone! (Hence, shark habits! Thank you, Robb Wolf, for this term.)

More importantly, shark habits have a profound impact on **mental health**. They remove friction. They clear space.

For the past few decades, I've discussed in depth how *shark habits*—simple, immediate, one-time decisions—can radically improve physical health. You know the list: see your doctor, visit the dentist, and see the eye doctor. At the end of the visit, they always ask if you want to schedule the next appointment. Your answer:

Yes.

Shark habits work. They support health, longevity, fitness, and performance.

Shark Habits and Longevity

One day at the Pacifica Barbell Club, Dick Notmeyer asked me a question. Now, with Dick, you had to understand: when he asked something, he usually already had the answer.

"Danny," he said, "by percentage, what do you think are the keys to a long life?"

He went on to break it down like this:

- **50% Genetics** – Some families just live long. You probably know someone who made it to 105 on cigarettes and moonshine.

- **40% Lifestyle** – The part we can improve—or ruin.

- **10% Luck** – Right place, right time. Or not.

The secret to longevity might be as simple as: **Don't die.** Sounds flippant, but there's wisdom in it.

Once you're past 55, nutritional tweaks matter less than **not breaking**. A bad fall in the shower is more life-changing than your choice between broccoli and kale. After midlife, your priorities shift: safety, balance, and mobility.

In *Spring Chicken*, Bill Gifford backs this up:

- Caloric restriction improves lifespan.

- Intermittent fasting is a simpler path to the same goal.

- Just **100 minutes of exercise a week** can add **seven years** to your life.

- Red wine, coffee, and a few smart supplements may help.

So, again: **Don't die.**

That leads to my corollary of Coach Maughan's advice to the college track team (*"Make yourself a slave to good habits)*:

Be a slave to shark habits.

Clear the clutter. Check the box. Remove the friction.

Think in **imperative sentences**:

- Go!
- Call!
- Do!

Hollywood knows the power of the imperative:

"Leave the gun. Take the cannoli." – *The Godfather*

"Go ahead, make my day." – *Sudden Impact*

"Fezzik, tear his arms off." – *The Princess Bride*

Shark habits are about *removing decisions*. Put the right systems in place once and let them run.

Pirate Maps for Ongoing Change

Once your shark habits are in place, you'll want a guide to stay on course. That's where **pirate maps** come in.

Pat Flynn coined the term. Think of a pirate map like this:

A treasure map isn't valuable because it's 100 pages long. It's valuable because it shows a clear path from A to B.

A pirate map is a simple, often single-page plan. Clear, direct, actionable. It works for fitness, finance, relationships—almost anything.

As Warren Buffett said in AARP Magazine (June/July 2016) about financial fitness:

- Hold cash for emergencies—and opportunities.
- Buy and hold.
- Embrace the boring.
- Stick with what you know.

Wisdom echoes across fields.

I learned a great summary of this decades ago:

Don't over-paper things.

The more words, the less impact.

How to Not Over-Paper Lifting

People want 500-page manuals for "eating clean." They want multi-volume tomes on "getting in shape."

But strength? That's easy.

If you want to get stronger: **Lift weights.**

Here is an amazing method:

One-Two-Three
Pick a big lift from each fundamental human movement:

- Push: bench press or military press

- Pull: pull-up
- Squat: front or back squat
- Hinge: deadlift
- Loaded carry: suitcase carry (just do these at the end and don't worry about reps)

Use a weight you can do for five reps. That's usually around 80% of your max. Perform:

- 1 rep, rest
- 2 reps, rest
- 3 reps, rest

That's six quality reps. Do three rounds for a quick day, five for a tough one. That's 18 to 30 total reps, all solid.

Key rule: **Never miss. Never chase fatigue.**

Dominate each set. Make the load feel light. Progress by adding a little over time.

There! I just gave you a program you can explore for years. Sleep for recovery, eat for nutrition.

And…nobody wants this! It's not Spartan or Warrior or whatever enough to sell, but it works.

Pirate Maps in Practice

Here's one of Pat Flynn's best pirate maps for daily living:

- Start the day by expressing gratitude.

- Occasionally, skip breakfast.
- Strength train 3–5 days a week. Get sweaty 2–3 times a week.
- Walk more than you drive. Take the stairs. Park far.
- Stretch what's tight.
- Develop a sleep ritual.
- Train consistently. Add variety for plateaus. Add randomness for fun.

That's it. That's the map.

"Walk five paces north from the palm tree next to the red rock, dig six feet, find treasure."

Even cookbooks follow pirate map logic—five-ingredient meals, slow cooker prep, one-pot dinners. Anything that benefits from repeatability benefits from pirate maps.

Of course, many will say: "That's too simple."

But I say: **Let's keep it that way.**

Chapter Thirteen

What Is an Elite Coach?

This is who we are.

An elite coach isn't just someone with a whistle and a clipboard. Elite coaching involves clarity, decisiveness, restraint, and principle-based execution. In my experience, the very best coaches share five essential traits:

1. The Elite Coach Understands Cost-to-Benefit Ratios

In the mid-1980s, I walked into our first department meeting of the year. I was emotionally prepared for a total waste of time. Our department head—famous for telling us the same thing over and over—had a quick announcement:

"Dan, we need you to teach senior economics this year."

Three days before school started, I was given a class dreaded by both students and faculty. So, I did what any coach would do—I went to the library.

Like most of us, I knew nothing about economics. But teaching that class turned out to be the best coaching experience of my life.

At first, I stayed just a couple of days ahead of the students. However, I quickly fell in love with the subject. Every lecture and discussion exploded with relevance. The concept that stuck with me most was the

cost-to-benefit ratio, and it became the cornerstone of my coaching, teaching, and life philosophy.

I often joke about the "Three Fs": **Fitness, Finance, and Relationships**. People sometimes wrinkle their noses at that, but these three areas are universal, and the cost-to-benefit ratio applies to all of them.

"Little and often over the long haul" beats quick fixes every time. Sure, you can take shortcuts—drugs for abs, get-rich-quick schemes, psychological manipulation—but long-term, they fail.

Cost-to-benefit ratios are straightforward: **every decision has both upsides and downsides. Our job is to know the trade-offs.**

- Yes, we can do more. But do we get better?
- Yes, we can add more load. But do we get better?
- Yes, we can take more supplements. But do we get better?

That's the question. That's the ratio.

It's easy to forget this in a world obsessed with "more." But elite coaches live in this space, understanding that *more* isn't always *better*. It takes maturity and clarity to say: "No, that's enough."

2. The Elite Coach Understands That Enough Is Enough

Let me clear up something important: *Enough Is Enough* is **not** the title of that famous Donna Summer song—that was *No More Tears*. You're welcome.

But the sentiment is valid:

Enough is enough.

I can't go on, I can't go on, no more.
I want him out that door now!

There's truth in those lyrics.

Conditioning athletes is easy. Just run them into the ground—more sprints, more up-downs, more suffering. But that doesn't make them better. You can stretch until your athletes are Gumby, but that rarely improves performance.

Yes, you *can* do more. But at some point, you must say: **Enough is enough.**

The elite coach knows when to stop.

3. The Elite Coach Knows to Correct the Correctable

This concept, which I first encountered in John T. Reed's writings, has stayed with me ever since. He breaks life into two categories:

- **Correctable**: things you can improve
- **Zen**: things you cannot

In baseball, for example:

Correctable skills:

- Catching a fly ball
- Sliding properly
- Bunting
- Waiting for a good pitch

Zen skills:

- Hitting a baseball
- Throwing accurately
- Fielding a tough grounder

Focus on the correctable, and your team improves.

This applies across life. Think geometry: there are **given** traits you can't change, and **variables**, things you can improve.

Givens:

- Height
- Eye color
- Where you were born
- Your upbringing
- Your early beliefs

Correctables:

- Physique
- Dress
- Hairstyle
- Location
- Career choices

You can't control your height. But you can control how you dress to enhance your physique. You can control your posture, your grooming, and how you present yourself.

The elite coach guides athletes to correct what can be corrected—and doesn't waste energy on what can't.

4. The Elite Coach Understands the Coach-Athlete Enthusiasm/Energy Split

Not everyone agrees with this.

Many coaching workshops preach that *you*, the coach, must be a fireball of energy at every session. But I've always disagreed.

Yes, sometimes I must pick athletes up and dust them off. But I'm not going to be in the ring, on the field, or in the pool when it counts. The athlete must learn to generate their enthusiasm and focus.

I use a model I call **"The 10 Units."**

Together, the coach and athlete must contribute a total of 10 units of energy or enthusiasm.

- Early on, I might provide 8, while you give 2.
- Later, you're putting in 9, and I'm replying to your email with a 1.
- Often, it's 5 and 5.

It shifts depending on the moment, but the total is always 10. The goal is to build athletes who *own* the energy and motivation.

The elite coach helps build that internal engine.

5. "You Make Three Decisions a Year That Matter"

I travel frequently and often find myself in first or business class. I've sat next to senators, famous actors, a former presidential candidate (I didn't vote for him), and major business leaders.

Once, I shared a long flight with a man who had just sold his company for a billion dollars. We talked fitness, leadership, and performance. And I'll never forget this:

"You make three decisions a year that matter."

Decisions. A deceptively simple word with deep meaning.

The root of "decision"—*cid* or *cis*—means "to cut or kill." Think: homicide, suicide, scissors. A real decision cuts off all other options.

Most people don't make real decisions. They tinker. They tweak. They change fonts on a document and call it leadership.

But a **true** decision sounds like this:

"Folks, we're doing *this*."

And if someone raises a hand, you say:

"Put that hand down."

The elite coach knows when to make real decisions—and how to follow through without revisiting them endlessly.

When you decide, **decide**. And move forward.

Coaching as a Job, Career, or Calling

My daughter Kelly—now a teacher and mother—once told me the secret to happiness comes down to this question:

"Do you see your work as a job, a career, or a calling?"

I've met coaches who treat it as a **job.** They show up when practice starts, check their phones, and do the bare minimum. That's fine—sometimes we take jobs to pay bills. However, in the long term, it's not fulfilling.

Some treat coaching as a **career**—a path to money, recognition, and championships. That can be satisfying too, if that's what you value.

But for some of us, coaching is a **calling.** It goes beyond reps, drills, and games. It's about shaping lives, building people, and impacting the future.

The **elite coach understands all three**, but the best coaches help raise everyone to the level of a calling.

Chapter Fourteen

A Conclusion: That Feedback Loop

Here's a quick recap:

Setting goals and doing assessments creates a **feedback loop**—one that looks a lot like a sideways figure eight.

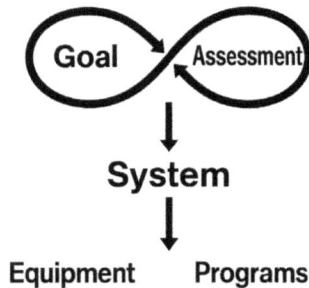

```
    ┌──────────┐
  Goal  →  Assessment
    └──────────┘
         │
         ▼
      System
         │
         ▼
  Equipment   Programs
```

It begins the moment someone asks, "What do you want?" or "What's your goal?" From that point, we sift through the near-infinite options available to the human person in this era of possibility.

Completing an **Assessment** provides even more clarity. It tells us what needs attention *right now*. Often, addressing that first need is the fastest route to the stated goal. Maybe we add new tools or new foods or new ideas. Assess them and remember:

- **A Grades** are magic. Find them. Cultivate them.

- **B Grades** are your foundation. Respect them.

- **C Grades** are experiments. Stay curious.
- **F Grades** are red flags. Walk away.

In training and in life:

Grow the As.

Conclusion

Health is about the inside. Fitness is about what you can do. Coaching is about navigating both. And living well—truly well—is about honoring the distinctions and working at the intersections.

So breathe deeply. Smile. Train. Assess. Eat like an adult. Get your sleep.

As we get close to our goal, a new challenge appears—we assess again—and the cycle continues. This loop will run for the entire life of the trainee.

The process is simple:

1. Do what is needed.
2. Follow an appropriate program.
3. Finish the program.
4. Reassess.

And the program often looks something like this:

- Stretch what is tightening: pecs, biceps, hip flexors, hamstrings *(from Vlad Janda)*.
- Strengthen what is weakening: glutes, abs, delts, triceps *(from Vlad Janda)*.

- Walk more. Sleep deep. Drink water. *(My mom)*
- Eat like an adult (*my instructions to practically every client*).
- Seek mastery (*from George Leonard*).

Let's finish with this important point:

"Let success happen."

There is no one more successful than the person striving for a worthy goal.

I hope you can guide your clients on this journey.

About Dan John

Dan John has spent more than sixty years lifting heavy things and trying to figure out why people make fitness so complicated. A former All-American discus thrower, Highland Games athlete, and Olympic lifter, Dan somehow turned throwing stuff and picking up iron into a career as a coach, teacher, and author.

He's written books like *Intervention*, *Can You Go?*, and *Now What?*, each one trying (again) to answer the age-old question: "Why aren't people doing the simple stuff that actually works?" Known for distilling complex training ideas into plain English, often with a story about coaching, parenting, or his own spectacular mistakes, Dan travels the world teaching workshops that blend humor, insight, and a healthy dose of common sense.

When he's not coaching or writing, you'll find him in Utah, gardening, lifting, reading, and trying to keep up with his grandkids, who've already outpaced his speed but haven't quite beaten his deadlift. Yet.

"Never Let Go"